M000034407

Sirtfood Diet Cookbook

Activate Your Skinny Gene and Burn Fat Fast With These 50+ Mouthwatering and Tasty Vegan, Carnivorous, and Vegetarian Recipes

AIDAN MATTEN

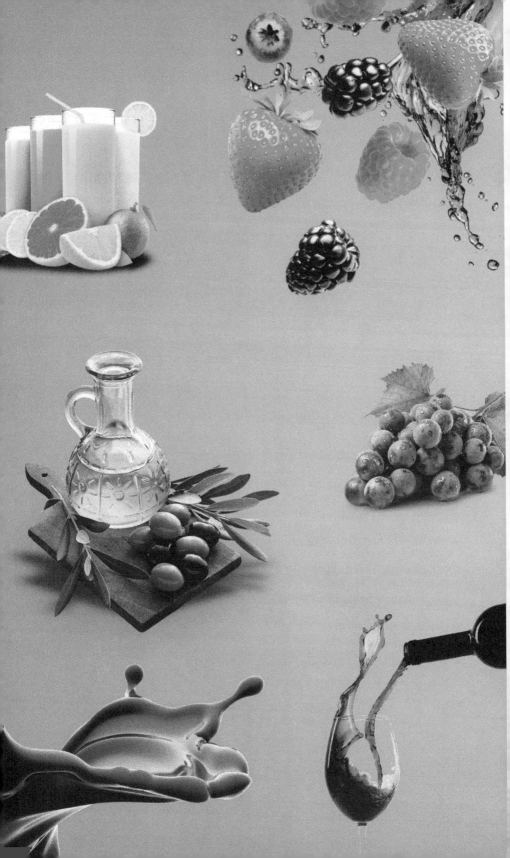

Table of Contents

INTRODUCTION 9

1. Salmon & Kale Omelet 11
2. Chilaquiles with Gochujang 13
3. Twice Baked Breakfast Potatoes 16
4. Vegan Thai Green Curry 19
5. Indian Yellow Curry 22
6. Tuna Salad in Red Chicory 24
7. Buckwheat Porridge 26
8. Nutty Green Beans 28
9. Rosemary Endives 30
10. Italian Veggie Salsa 32
11. Black Bean Salsa 34
12. Corn Spread 36
13. Mushroom Dip 38
14. Chocolate Waffles 40
15. Eggs with Kale 43
16. Chocolate Sauce 45
17. Hot Sauce 47
18. Paleo Breakfast Salad with Egg 49
19. Caesar Dressing 51
20. Chicken, Kale, & Carrot Salad 53
21. Fried Cauliflower Rice 56
22. Mediterranean Paleo Pizza 58
23. Fried Chicken and Broccolini 61
24. Braised Leek with Pine Nuts 63
25. Mussels in Red Wine Sauce 65
26. Roast Balsamic Vegetables 67
27. Ginger Prawn Stir-Fry 69
28. Chicken with Mole Salad 71
29. Honey Chili Nuts 73
30. Cauliflower Nachos 75
31. Tofu Smoothie 77
32. Grape Smoothie 79
33. Kale and Cucumber Smoothie 80
34. Mozzarella Cauliflower Bars 82
35. Walnut and Date Bites 84
36. Sirt Energy Balls 85

37. Hot Chicory & Nut Salad 87
38. Tuscan Bean Stew 89
39. Sirtfood Cauliflower Couscous and Turkey Steak 91
40. Chicken Thighs with Tomato Spinach Sauce 93
41. Chicken with Mole Salad 95
42. Honey Chili Squash 97
43. Turkey Escalope with Cauliflower Couscous 99
44. Strawberry Arugula Salad 101
45. Serrano Ham & Rocket Arugula 103
46. Tomato & Goat's Cheese Pizza 105
47. Banana Dessert 107
48. Salad with Roasted Carrots 109
49. Salmon with Capers and Lemon 111
50. Pasta Salad 113
51. Pine and Sunflower Seed Rolls 115
52. Tofu with Cauliflower 118
53. Sweet and Sour Pan 121
54. Vegetarian Curry 123
55. Spiced Burger 125

Introduction

A re you currently on a diet that promises lots of results but offers practically none? Do you want a unique approach that has shown good results? Well, the sirtfood diet is that one meal plan that can guarantee prominent weight loss in just a few weeks.

Who knew that a diet named Sirtfood would become the new buzzword for the year? Well, as much as the word "sirtfood" sounds unique and different, the diet itself has been surprising people around the world due to its amazing health benefits. The Sirtfood diet is taking over the stage as one of the most tempting diet regimens created for regulated, balanced, and healthy weight loss. The Sirtfood diet is also known as one of the most appreciated diets in inclusive celebrity circles, created by two nutritionists based in the UK. Why is the diet called the Sirtfood diet and how are sirtuins beneficial to your body? You will find the answers to these and more questions as you are entering the world of sirtfoods and plant-based protein. We have created a compilation of Sirtfood diet-friendly recipes to help you get started with your weight loss regimen; you will also find ultimate grocery lists and top Sirtfood ingredients to shop for before your three-week journey.

If you are looking for a diet that helps attain your weight loss and fitness objectives without compromising your taste buds, try the Sirtfood diet. It teaches healthy eating habits and increases your body's natural metabolism by activating a group of proteins known as "sirtuins".

The Sirtfood diet was created by the famous duo of health consultants and celebrity nutritionists Aidan Goggins and Glen Matten. Instead of purely concentrating on weight loss, this diet encourages healthy eating patterns. The secret to weight loss, enhancement of your body's natural mechanism and its healing powers is to consume foods rich in sirtuins. This is not a fad diet; it activates your body's natural fat-burning mechanism, promotes weight loss, improves your immune function, is incredibly simple to follow, and leaves you feeling energetic. A great thing about this diet is that you can achieve all the benefits it offers without depriving yourself of the foods you enjoy. TV chef Lorraine Pascal, model Jodie Kidd, champion boxer David Haye, and beloved music icon Adele follow the Sirtfood diet. From red wine and dark chocolate to coffee, you can add different delicious ingredients to this diet.

In this book, you will discover several mouthwatering Sirtfood diet recipes. Enjoy!

1. Salmon & Kale Omelet

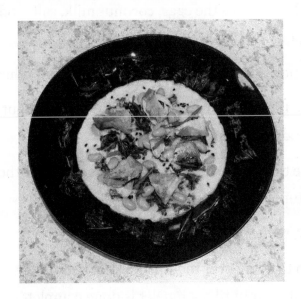

Preparation time: 10 minutes

Cooking time: 7 minutes

Servings: 4

Ingredients:

- 6 eggs

- 2 tablespoons unsweetened almond milk

- Salt and ground black pepper, to taste

- 2 tablespoons olive oil

- 4 ounces smoked salmon, cut into bite-sized chunks

- 2 cup fresh kale, tough ribs removed and chopped finely

- 4 scallions, chopped finely

Directions:

1. In a bowl, place the eggs, coconut milk, salt, and black pepper, and beat well. Set aside.

2. In a non-stick wok, heat the oil over medium heat.

3. Place the egg mixture evenly and cook for about 30 seconds, without stirring.

4. Place the salmon kale and scallions on top of the egg mixture evenly.

5. Now, reduce heat to low.

6. With the lid, cover the wok and cook for about 4–5 minutes, or until the omelet is done completely.

7. Uncover the wok and cook for about 1 minute.

8. Carefully, transfer the omelet onto a serving plate and serve.

Nutrition: calories 212, fat 15, fiber 4, carbs 5, protein 14

2. Chilaquiles with Gochujang

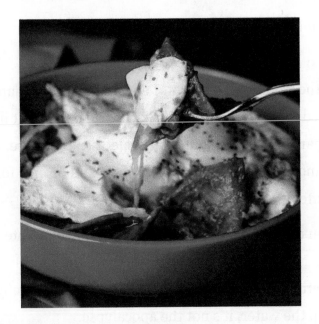

Preparation time: 30 minutes

Cooking time: 20 minutes

Servings: 2

Ingredients:

- One dried ancho chile

- 2 cups of water

- 1 cup squashed tomatoes

- Two cloves of garlic

- One teaspoon genuine salt

- 1/2 tablespoons gochujang

- 5 to 6 cups tortilla chips

- Three large eggs

- One tablespoon olive oil

Directions:

1. Get the water to heat a pot. I cheated marginally and heated the water in an electric pot and emptied it into the pan. There's no sound unrivaled strategy here. Add the ancho chile to the bubbled water and drench for 15 minutes to give it an opportunity to stout up.

2. When completed, use tongs or a spoon to extricate chile. Make sure to spare the water for the sauce! Nonetheless, on the off chance that you incidentally dump the water, it's not the apocalypse.

3. Mix the doused chile, 1 cup of saved high temp water, squashed tomatoes, garlic, salt, and gochujang until smooth.

4. Empty the sauce into a large dish and warm over medium for 4 to 5 minutes. Mood killer the heat and include the tortilla chips. Mix the chips to cover with the sauce. In a different skillet, shower a teaspoon of oil and fry an egg on top, until the whites have settled. Plate the egg and cook the remainder of the eggs. If you are phenomenal at performing various tasks, you can likely sear the eggs while you heat the red sauce. I am not precisely so capable.

5. Top the chips with the seared eggs, cotija, hacked cilantro, jalapeños, onions, and avocado. Serve right away.

Nutrition: calories 487, fat 19, fiber 4, carbs 23, protein 13

3. Twice Baked Breakfast Potatoes

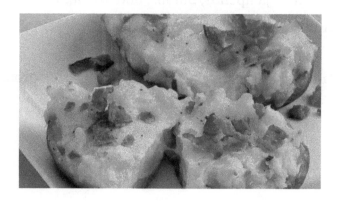

Preparation time: 1 hour 10 minutes

Cooking time: 1 hour

Servings: 2

Ingredients:

- 2 medium reddish brown potatoes, cleaned and pricked with a fork everywhere

- 2 tablespoons unsalted spread

- 3 tablespoons overwhelming cream

- 4 rashers cooked bacon

- 4 large eggs

- ½ cup destroyed cheddar

- Daintily cut chives

- Salt and pepper to taste

Directions:

1. Preheat oven to 400°F.

2. Spot potatoes straightforwardly on the oven rack in the focal point of the grill and prepare for 30 to 45 min.

3. Take out and permit potatoes to cool for around 15 minutes.

4. Cut every potato down the middle longwise and burrow every half out, scooping the potato centered into a blending bowl.

5. Add margarine and cream to the potato and pound into a single unit until smooth — season with salt and pepper and mix.

6. Spread a portion of the potato blend into the base of each emptied potato skin and sprinkle with one tablespoon cheddar (you may make them remain pounded potato left to snack on).

7. Add one rasher bacon to every half and top with a raw egg.

8. Spot potatoes onto a heating sheet and come back to the appliance.

9. Lower oven temperature to 375°F and heat potatoes until egg whites are simply set and yolks are as yet runny.

10. Top every potato with a sprinkle of the rest of the cheddar, season with salt and pepper, and finish with cut chives.

Nutrition: calories 642, fat 35, fiber 4, carbs 9, protein 30

4. Vegan Thai Green Curry

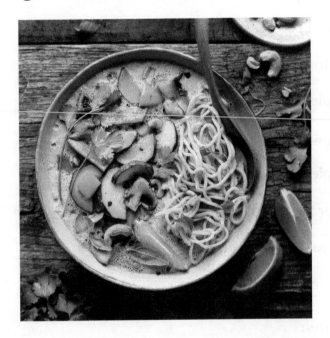

Preparation Time: 45 minutes

Cooking Time: 4 hours

Servings: 8

Ingredients:

- 2 pieces of green chilies

- 1 piece Onion

- 1 clove Garlic

- 1 teaspoon fresh ginger (grated)

- 25 g fresh coriander

- 1 teaspoon ground caraway

- 1 piece Lime (juice)

- 1 teaspoon Coconut oil

- 500 ml Coconut milk

- 1 piece Zucchini

- 1 piece Broccoli

- 1 piece Red pepper

- For the cauliflower rice:

- 1 teaspoon Coconut oil

- 1 piece Cauliflower

Directions:

1. For the cauliflower rice, cut the cauliflower into florets and place them in the food processor. Pulse briefly until the rice has formed. Put aside.

2. Cut the green peppers, onions, garlic, fresh ginger, and coriander into large pieces and combine with the caraway seeds and the juice of 1 lime in a food processor or blender and mix to an even paste.

3. Heat a pan over medium heat with a teaspoon of coconut oil and gently fry the pasta. Deglaze with coconut milk and add to the slow cooker.

4. Cut the zucchini into pieces, the broccoli in florets, the peppers into cubes, and put in the slow cooker. Simmer

for 4 hours. Briefly heat the cauliflower rice in 1 teaspoon of coconut oil, season with a little salt and pepper in a pan over medium heat.

Nutrition: calories 192, fat 10, fiber 6, carbs 23, protein 7

5. Indian Yellow Curry

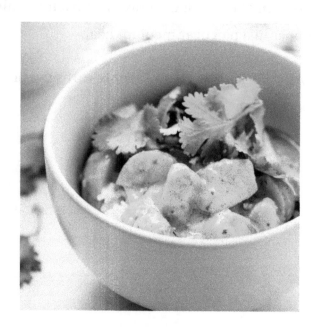

Preparation Time: 45 minutes

Cooking Time: 4 hours

Servings: 8

Ingredients:

- 2 pieces Onion

- 1 clove Garlic

- 300 g Chicken breast

- 2 teaspoon Coconut oil

- 1 tablespoon Curry powder

- 1 teaspoon fresh ginger

- 1 teaspoon dried turmeric

- Laos 1 tsp.

- 500 ml Coconut milk

For the salad:
- 250 g Iceberg lettuce

- 1/2 pieces Cucumber

- 2 pieces Red peppers

- 25 g Dried coriander

Directions:

1. Heat a saucepan over medium heat and let the coconut oil melt. Finely, chop onions and clove of garlic. Put in the pot and add the herbs, deglaze with the coconut milk and stir well.

2. Cut the chicken into cubes and add to the slow cooker along with the curry sauce and let it cook for 4 hours.

3. Cut iceberg lettuce, spread cucumber, and bell pepper cubes over it, and season with the coriander. Serve the salad with the curry.

Nutrition: calories 122, fat 40, fiber 14, carbs 48, protein 75

6. Tuna Salad in Red Chicory

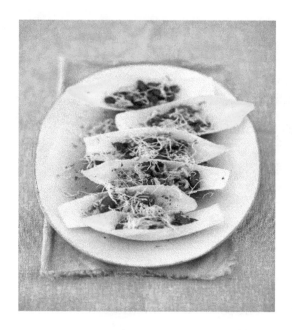

Preparation Time: 10 minutes

Cooking Time: 5 minutes

Servings: 2

Ingredients:

- 4 pieces Red chicory

- 160 g Tuna (tin)

- 1 piece Orange

- 1 tablespoon fresh parsley (finely chopped.)

- 5 pieces Radish

- 1 / 2 TL Apple cider vinegar

Directions:

1. Drain the tuna.

2. Cut the orange into wedges and cut them into small pieces.

3. Cut radishes into small pieces.

4. Mix all the ingredients (except the red chicory) in a small bowl. Season with salt and pepper

5. Spread the tuna salad on the red chicory leaves.

Nutrition: calories 243, fat 4, fiber 27, carbs 5, protein 41

7. Buckwheat Porridge

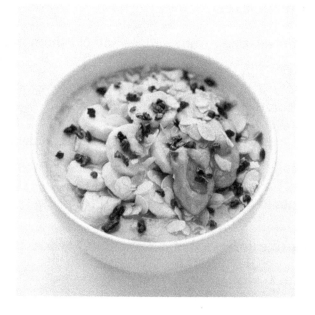

Preparation time: 10 minutes

Cooking time: 15 minutes

Servings: 2

Ingredients:

- 1 cup buckwheat (rinsed)

- 1 cup unsweetened almond milk

- 1 cup water

- ½ teaspoon ground cinnamon

- ½ teaspoon vanilla extract

- 1–2 tablespoons raw honey

- ¼ cup fresh blueberries

Directions:

1. In a pan, add all the ingredients (except honey and blueberries) over medium-high heat and bring to a boil.

2. Now, reduce the heat to low and simmer, covered for about 10 minutes.

3. Stir in the honey and remove from the heat.

4. Set aside, covered for about 5 minutes.

5. With a fork, fluff the mixture, and transfer it into serving bowls.

6. Top with blueberries and serve.

Nutrition: calories 352, fat 5, fiber 4, carbs 4, protein 13

8. Nutty Green Beans

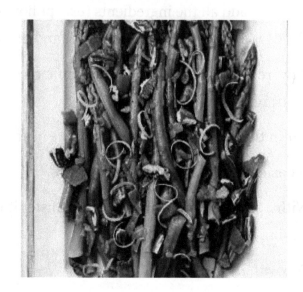

Preparation time: 10 minutes

Cooking time: 25 minutes

Servings: 2

Ingredients:

- 2 tbsps. each chunky-style peanut butter

- 2 tbsps. sherry

- 2 tbsps. oyster sauce

- 1 garlic clove (minced)

- 1/2 tsp. minced pared ginger root

- 2 c. cooked frozen French-style green beans (hot)

Directions:

1. In a small saucepan, combine peanut butter, sherry, oyster sauce, garlic, and ginger; bring to a boil.

2. Reduce heat and let simmer, continually stirring until mixture is creamy about 1 minute.

3. Pour peanut butter mixture over hot green beans and serve immediately.

Nutrition: calories 112, fat 5, fiber 4, carbs 5, protein 4

9. Rosemary Endives

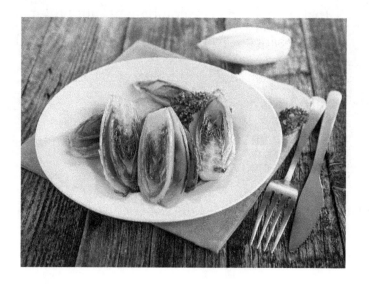

Preparation time: 10 minutes

Cooking time: 30 minutes

Servings: 2

Ingredients:

- 2 tbsps. Olive oil

- 1 tsp. dried rosemary

- 2 halved endives

- ¼ tsp. black pepper

- ½ tsp. turmeric powder

Directions:

1. In a baking pan, combine the endives with the oil and the other ingredients, toss gently, introduce in the oven and bake at 400°F for 20 minutes. Divide between plates and serve.

Nutrition: calories 112, fat 5, fiber 4, carbs 5, protein 4

10.   Italian Veggie Salsa

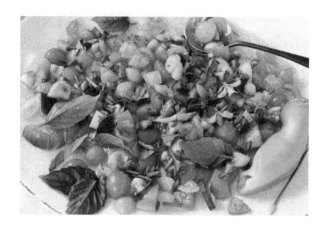

Preparation time: 10 minutes

Cooking time: 10 minutes

Servings: 4

Ingredients:

- 2 red bell peppers cut into medium wedges

- 3 zucchinis (sliced)

- ½ cup garlic (minced)

- 2 tablespoons olive oil

- A pinch of black pepper

- 1 teaspoon Italian seasoning

Directions:

1. Heat a pan with the oil over medium-high heat, add bell peppers and zucchini, toss and cook for 5 minutes.

2. Add garlic, black pepper, and Italian seasoning, toss, cook for 5 minutes more, divide into small cups, and serve as a snack.

3. Enjoy!

Nutrition: Calories 132, Fat 3, Fiber 3, Carbs 7, Protein 4

11. Black Bean Salsa

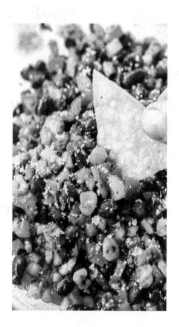

Preparation time: 10 minutes

Cooking time: 0 minutes

Servings: 6

Ingredients:

- 1 tablespoon coconut aminos

- ½ teaspoon cumin (ground)

- 1 cup canned black beans, no-salt-added, drained and rinsed

- 1 cup salsa

- 6 cups romaine lettuce leaves (torn)

- ½ cup avocado, peeled, pitted, and cubed

Directions:

1. In a bowl, combine the beans with the aminos, cumin, salsa, lettuce, and avocado, toss, divide into small bowls, and serve as a snack.

2. Enjoy!

Nutrition: Calories 181 Fat 4 Fiber 7 Carbs 14 Protein 7

12. Corn Spread

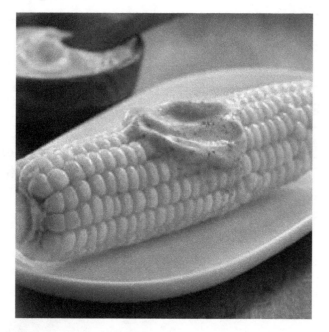

Preparation time: 10 minutes

Cooking time: 10 minutes

Servings: 6

Ingredients:

- 30 ounces canned corn (drained)

- 2 green onions (chopped)

- ½ cup coconut cream

- 1 jalapeno (chopped)

- ½ teaspoon chili powder

Directions:

1. In a small pan, combine the corn with green onions, jalapeno, and chili powder, stir, bring to a simmer, cook over medium heat for 10 minutes, leave aside to cool down, add coconut cream, stir well, divide into small bowls and serve as a spread.

2. Enjoy!

Nutrition: Calories 192, Fat 5, Fiber 10, Carbs 11, Protein 8

13. Mushroom Dip

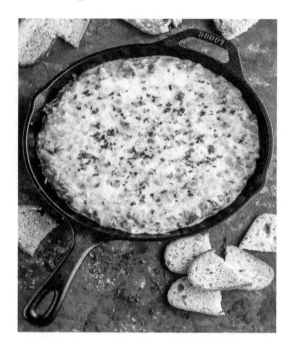

Preparation time: 10 minutes

Cooking time: 20 minutes

Servings: 6

Ingredients:

- 1 cup yellow onion (chopped)

- 3 garlic cloves (minced)

- 1-pound mushrooms (chopped)

- 28 ounces tomato sauce (no-salt-added)

- Black pepper to the taste

Directions:

1. Put the onion in a pot, add garlic, mushrooms, black pepper, and tomato sauce, stir, cook over medium heat for 20 minutes, leave aside to cool down, divide into small bowls and serve.

2. Enjoy!

Nutrition: Calories 215, Fat 4, Fiber 7, Carbs 3, Protein 7

14. Chocolate Waffles

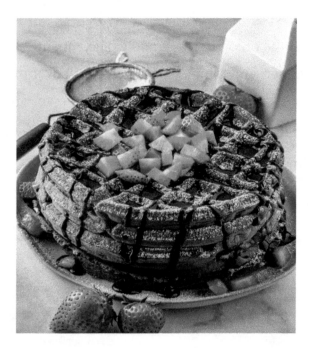

Preparation time: 15 minutes

Cooking time: 24 minutes

Servings: 8

Ingredients:

- 2 cups unsweetened almond milk

- 1 tablespoon fresh lemon juice

- 1 cup buckwheat flour

- ½ cup cacao powder

- ¼ cup flaxseed meal

- 1 teaspoon baking soda

- 1 teaspoon baking powder

- ¼ teaspoons kosher salt

- 2 large eggs

- ½ cup coconut oil (melted)

- ¼ cup dark brown sugar

- 2 teaspoons vanilla extract

- 2 ounces unsweetened dark chocolate (chopped roughly)

Directions:

1. In a bowl, add the almond milk and lemon juice and mix well.

2. Set aside for about 10 minutes.

3. In a bowl, place buckwheat flour, cacao powder, flaxseed meal, baking soda, baking powder, and salt, and mix well.

4. In the bowl of the almond milk mixture, place the eggs, coconut oil, brown sugar, and vanilla extract, and beat until smooth.

5. Now, place the flour mixture and beat until smooth.

6. Gently, fold in the chocolate pieces.

7. Preheat the waffle iron and then grease it.

8. Place the desired amount of the mixture into the preheated waffle iron and cook for about 3 minutes, or until golden brown.

9. Repeat with the remaining mixture.

Nutrition: calories 292, fat 22, fiber 4, carbs 2, protein 7

15. Eggs with Kale

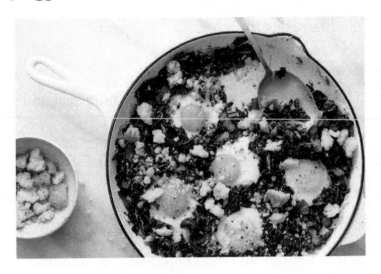

Preparation time: 15 minutes

Cooking time: 25 minutes

Servings: 4

Ingredients:

- 2 tablespoons olive oil

- 1 yellow onion (chopped)

- 2 garlic cloves (minced)

- 1 cup tomatoes (chopped)

- ½ pound fresh kale (tough ribs removed and chopped)

- 1 teaspoon ground cumin

- ¼ teaspoon red pepper flakes (crushed)

- Salt and ground black pepper (to taste)

- 4 eggs

- 2 tablespoons fresh parsley (chopped)

Directions:

1. Heat the oil in a large wok over medium heat and sauté the onion for about 4–5 minutes.

2. Add garlic and sauté for about 1 minute.

3. Add the tomatoes, spices, salt, and black pepper, and cook for about 2–3 minutes, stirring frequently.

4. Stir in the kale and cook for about 4–5 minutes.

5. Carefully, crack eggs on top of the kale mixture.

6. With the lid, cover the wok and cook for about 10 minutes, or until the desired doneness of eggs.

7. Serve hot with the garnishing of parsley.

Nutrition: calories 112, fat 5, fiber 4, carbs 5, protein 4

16.Chocolate Sauce

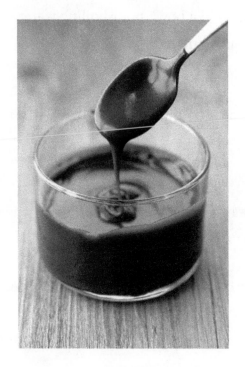

Preparation Time: 10 minutes

Cooking Time: 10 minutes

Servings: 2 cups

Ingredients:

- 75 g Cocoa powder

- 250 ml Coconut milk (can)

- 95 pieces Dates

- 3 tablespoon Coconut oil

- ½ teaspoon Vanilla extract

- 1 pinch Salt

Directions:

1. Put the dates in a bowl, pour boiling water over them and let them stand for 10 minutes.

2. Drain the dates.

3. Heat the coconut milk and coconut oil in a pan.

4. Place all the ingredients in a blender and puree into an even sauce.

5. Add some hot water if you think the sauce is too thick. (Mix them again if you add water).

Nutrition: calories 254, fat 45, fiber 43, carbs 56, protein 28

17. Hot Sauce

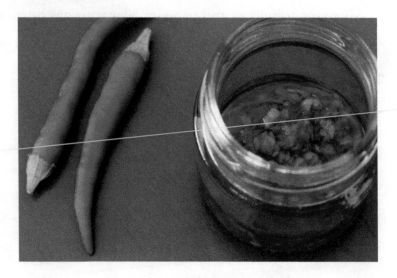

Preparation Time: 10 minutes

Cooking Time: 15 minutes

Servings: 1 cup

Ingredients:

- 2 pieces Tomato

- 2 pieces Red peppers

- 10 cloves Garlic

- 2 pieces Red pepper

- 250 ml White wine vinegar

- 2 tablespoons Olive oil

- 1 tablespoon Honey

- 1 tablespoon Celtic sea salt

Directions:

1. Singe the tomatoes and peppers over your gas burner. (Or in the oven at 220°C if you don't have a gas burner)

2. Let cool down.

3. Cut the paprika into pieces and remove the stones.

4. Heat a pan and roast the garlic (without oil) for a few minutes. Let cool down.

5. Clean the peppers, remove the seeds if necessary.

6. Put the tomatoes, garlic, and peppers in a blender.

7. Add 125 ml of water and puree well.

8. Pour the mixture into a saucepan and add the oil, honey, salt, and vinegar. Bring the mixture to a boil. Turn the heat down as soon as it boils and let it simmer for 5 minutes.

9. Let cool and check if the sauce still needs salt.

10. Put the sauce in a glass and let it rest in the fridge for 2 days. Thereupon she will soon burst with taste.

11. Before use; take a bowl and put a fine sieve on it. Pour the sauce over the sieve and press as far as possible with the convex side of the spoon.

12. You can throw away the residues remaining in the sieve.

Nutrition: calories 338, fat 28, fiber 4, carbs 45, protein 6

18.Paleo Breakfast Salad with Egg

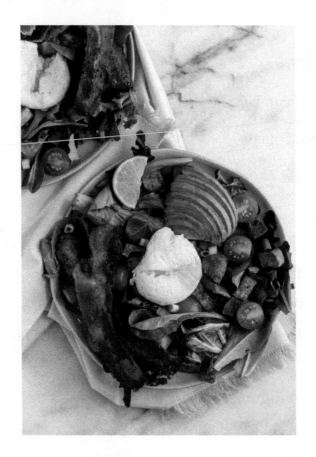

Preparation Time: 10 minutes

Cooking Time: 5 minutes

Servings: 2 - 3
Ingredients:

- 1 teaspoon Ghee

- 2 pieces Egg

- 1 hand Spinach

- ½ pieces Red bell pepper

- ¼ pieces Onion

- 50 g Carrot

- 50 g Cucumber

- 1 piece Tomato

- ½ pieces Avocado

Directions:
1. Slice the onion, cut the bell pepper into strips, cut the cucumber and avocado into cubes, grate the carrot, and cut the tomato into wedges.

2. Melt the ghee in a pan over medium heat and beat the eggs into the pan.

3. In the meantime, prepare the salad by putting all the remaining ingredients on a plate.

4. Remove the eggs from the pan when the egg yolk is still a little soft, this looks like a delicious dressing! (Or if you prefer a well-fried egg, drizzle your salad with some olive oil as a dressing).

5. Season with salt and pepper.

Nutrition: calories 112, fat 5, fiber 4, carbs 5, protein 4

19.Caesar Dressing

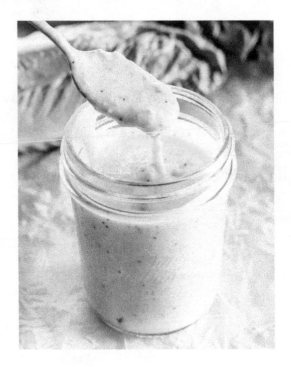

Preparation Time: 10 minutes

Cooking Time: 5 minutes

Servings: 1 cup

Ingredients:

- 250 ml Olive oil

- 2 tablespoons Lemon juice

- 4 pieces Anchovy fillet

- 2 tablespoon Mustard yellow

- 1 clove Garlic

- 1/2 teaspoon salt

- ½ teaspoon Black pepper

Directions:

1. Remove the peel from the garlic and chop it finely.

2. Put all ingredients in a blender and puree evenly.

3. This dressing can be kept in the fridge for about 3 days.

Nutrition: calories 71, fat 4, fiber 3, carbs 5, protein 8

20. Chicken, Kale, & Carrot Salad

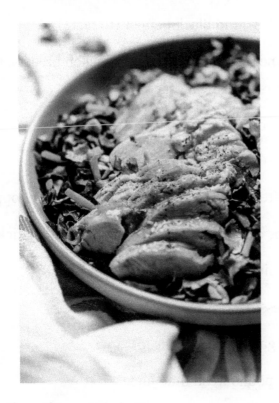

Preparation time: 15 minutes

Cooking time: 18 minutes

Servings: 4

Ingredients:

For Chicken:

- 1 teaspoon dried thyme

- ½ teaspoon garlic powder

- ½ teaspoon onion powder

- ¼ teaspoon cayenne pepper

- ¼ teaspoon ground turmeric

- Salt and ground black pepper (to taste)

- 2 (7-ounce) boneless, skinless chicken breasts, pounded into a ¾-inch thickness

- 1 tablespoon olive oil

For Salad:
- 5 cups fresh kale (tough ribs removed and chopped)

- 1½ cups carrots (peeled and cut into matchsticks)

- ¼ cup pine nuts

- For Dressing:

- 1 small garlic clove (minced)

- 2 tablespoons fresh lime juice

- 2 tablespoons extra-virgin olive oil

- 1 teaspoon raw honey

- ½ teaspoon Dijon mustard

Directions:

1. Preheat your oven to 425°F and line a baking dish with parchment paper.

2. For the chicken: in a bowl, mix the thyme, spices, salt, and black pepper.

3. Drizzle the chicken breasts with oil and then rub with spice mixture generously and drizzle with the oil.

4. Arrange the chicken breasts onto the prepared baking dish.

5. Bake for about 16–18 minutes.

6. Remove pan from oven, transfer chicken breasts onto a cutting board for about 5 minutes.

7. For the salad: place all ingredients in a salad bowl and mix.

8. For the dressing: place all ingredients in another bowl and beat until well combined.

9. Cut each chicken breast into desired sized slices.

10. Place the salad onto each serving plate and top each with chicken slices.

11. Drizzle with dressing and serve.

Nutrition: calories 312, fat 19, fiber 4, carbs 17, protein 25

21. Fried Cauliflower Rice

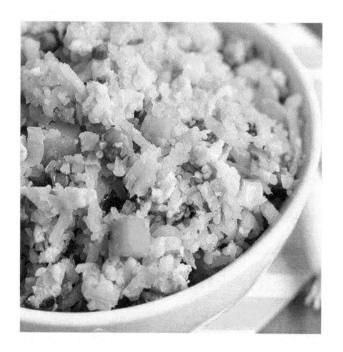

Preparation Time: 20 minutes

Cooking Time: 25 minutes

Servings: 4

Ingredients:

- 1 piece Cauliflower

- 2 tablespoon Coconut oil

- 1 piece Red onion

- 4 cloves Garlic

- 60 ml vegetable broth

- 1.5 cm fresh ginger

- 1 teaspoon Chili flakes

Directions:

1. Cut the cauliflower into small rice grains in a food processor.

2. Finely chop the onion, garlic, and ginger, cut the carrot into thin strips, dice the bell pepper and finely chop the herbs.

3. Melt 1 tablespoon of coconut oil in a pan and add half of the onion and garlic to the pan and fry briefly until translucent.

4. Add cauliflower rice and season with salt. Pour in the broth and stir everything until it evaporates and the cauliflower rice is tender.

5. Take the rice out of the pan and set it aside. Melt the rest of the coconut oil in the pan and add the remaining onions, garlic, ginger, carrots, and peppers.

6. Fry for a few minutes until the vegetables are tender. Season them with a little salt. Add the cauliflower rice again, heat the whole dish and add the lemon juice.

7. Garnish with pumpkin seeds and coriander before serving.

Nutrition: calories 252, fat 32, fiber 4, carbs 32, protein 10

22.   Mediterranean Paleo Pizza

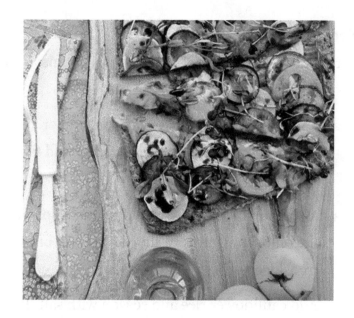

Preparation Time: 15 minutes

Cooking Time: 15 minutes

Servings: 3 - 4

Ingredients:

For the pizza crusts:

- 120 g Tapioca flour

- 1 teaspoon Celtic sea salt

- 2 tablespoon Italian spice mix

- 45 g Coconut flour

- 120 ml Olive oil (mild)

- Water (warm) 120 ml

- Egg (beaten) 1 piece

For covering:

- 2 pieces Tomato

- 2 tablespoon Olive oil (mild)

- 1 tablespoon Balsamic vinegar

Directions:

1. Preheat the oven to 190°C and line a baking sheet with parchment paper.

2. Cut the vegetables into thin slices.

3. Mix the tapioca flour with salt, Italian herbs, and coconut flour in a large bowl.

4. Pour in olive oil and warm water and stir well.

5. Then add the egg and stir until you get an even dough.

6. If the dough is too shrill, add 1 tablespoon of coconut flour at a time until it is the desired thickness. Always wait a few minutes before adding more coconut flour, as it will take some time to absorb the moisture. The intent is to get a soft, sticky dough.

7. Split the dough into two parts, and spread them in flat circles on the baking sheet (or make 1 large sheet of pizza as shown in the picture).

8. Bake in the oven for about 10 minutes.

9. Brush the pizza with tomato paste and spread the aubergines, zucchini, and tomato overlapping on the pizza.

10. Drizzle the pizza with olive oil and bake in the oven for another 10-15 minutes.

11. Drizzle balsamic vinegar over the pizza before serving.

Nutrition: calories 112, fat 5, fiber 4, carbs 5, protein 4

23.   Fried Chicken and Broccolini

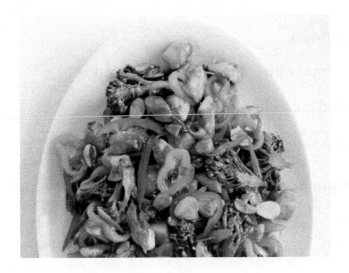

Preparation Time: 10 minutes

Cooking Time: 15 minutes

Servings: 5

Ingredients:

- 2 tablespoon Coconut oil

- 400g Chicken breast

- Bacon cubes 150g

- Broccolini 250g

Directions:

1. Cut the chicken into cubes.

2. Melt the coconut oil in a pan over medium heat and brown the chicken with the bacon cubes and cook through.

3. Season with chili flakes, salt, and pepper.

4. Add broccolini and fry.

5. Stack on a plate and enjoy!

Nutrition: calories 112, fat 5, fiber 4, carbs 5, protein 4

24. Braised Leek with Pine Nuts

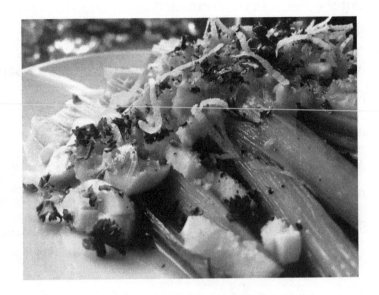

Preparation Time: 15 minutes

Cooking Time: 15 minutes

Servings: 4

Ingredients:

- 20 g Ghee

- 2 teaspoon Olive oil

- 2 pieces Leek

- 150 ml vegetable broth

- Fresh parsley

- 1 tablespoon fresh oregano

- 1 tablespoon Pine nuts (roasted)

Directions:

1. Cut the leek into thin rings and finely chop the herbs. Roast the pine nuts in a dry pan over medium heat.

2. Melt the ghee together with the olive oil in a large pan.

3. Cook the leek until golden brown for 5 minutes, stirring constantly.

4. Add the vegetable broth and cook for another 10 minutes until the leek is tender.

5. Stir in the herbs and sprinkle the pine nuts on the dish just before serving.

Nutrition: calories 189, fat 5, fiber 3, carbs 25, protein 4

25.   **Mussels in Red Wine Sauce**

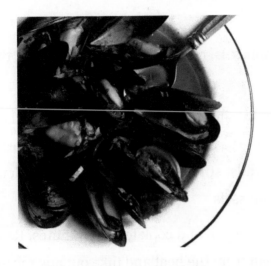

Preparation time: 5 Minutes

Cooking Time: 50 Minutes

Servings: 2

Ingredients:

- 800g 2lb mussels

- 2 x 400g 14 oz. tins of chopped tomatoes

- 25g 1oz butter

- 1 tablespoon fresh chives (chopped)

- 1 tablespoon fresh parsley (chopped)

- 1 bird's-eye chili (finely chopped)

- 4 cloves of garlic (crushed)

- 400 ml 14fl. oz. red wine

- Juice of 1 lemon

Directions:

1. Wash the mussels, remove their beards, and set them aside.

2. Heat the butter in a large saucepan and add in the red wine. Reduce the heat and add the parsley, chives, chili, and garlic whilst stirring. Add in the tomatoes, lemon juice, and mussels.

3. Cover the saucepan and cook for 2-3 minutes. Remove the saucepan from the heat and take out any mussels which haven't opened and discard them. Serve and eat immediately.

Nutrition: calories 362, fat 9, fiber 4, carbs 5, protein 36

26.   Roast Balsamic Vegetables

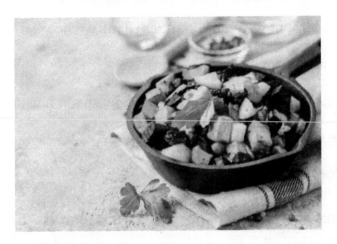

Preparation time: 5 Minutes

Cooking Time: 45 Minutes

Servings: 2

Ingredients:

- 4 tomatoes (chopped)

- 2 red onions (chopped)

- 3 sweet potatoes (peeled and chopped)

- 100g 3½ oz. red chicory or if unavailable (use yellow)

- 100g 3½ oz. kale (finely chopped)

- 300g 11oz potatoes (peeled and chopped)

- 5 stalks of celery (chopped)

- 1 bird's-eye chili (de-seeded and finely chopped)

- 2 tablespoons fresh parsley (chopped)

- 2 tablespoons fresh coriander cilantro (chopped)

- 3 tablespoons olive oil

- 2 tablespoons balsamic vinegar 1 teaspoon mustard

- Sea salt

- Freshly ground black pepper

Directions:

1. Place the olive oil, balsamic, mustard, parsley, and coriander cilantro into a bowl and mix well.

2. Toss all the remaining ingredients into the dressing and season with salt and pepper.

3. Transfer the vegetables to an ovenproof dish and cook in the oven at 400°F for 45 minutes.

Nutrition: calories 312, fat 10, fiber 4, carbs 29, protein 4

27.   Ginger Prawn Stir-Fry

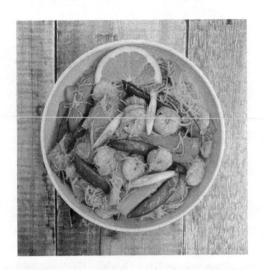

Preparation time: 5 Minutes

Cooking Time: 50 Minutes

Servings: 1

Ingredients:

- 6 prawns or shrimp (peeled and deveined)

- ½ packages of buckwheat noodles called Soba in Asian

- 5-6 leaves of kale (chopped)

- 1 cup of green beans (chopped)

- 5g lovage or celery leaves

- 1 garlic clove (finely chopped)

- 1 bird's eye chili (finely chopped)

- 1 tsp. fresh ginger (finely chopped)

- 2 stalks celery (chopped)

- ½ small red onion (chopped)

- 1 cup chicken stock or vegetable if you prefer

- 2 tbsp. soy sauce

- 2 tbsp. extra virgin olive oil

Directions:

1. Cook prawns in a bit of the oil and soy sauce until done and set aside (about 10-15 minutes).

2. Boil the noodles according to the directions (usually 6-8 minutes). Set aside.

3. Sauté the vegetables, then add the garlic, ginger, red onion, and chili in a bit of oil until tender and crunchy, but not mushy. Add the prawns, and noodles, and simmer low about 5-10 minutes past that point.

Nutrition: calories 112, fat 5, fiber 4, carbs 5, protein 4

28. Chicken with Mole Salad

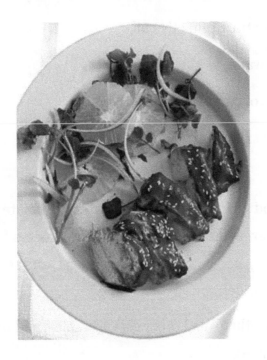

Preparation time: 5 Minutes

Cooking Time: 40 Minutes

Servings: 2

Ingredients:

- 1 skinned chicken breast

- 2 cups spinach (washed, dried, and torn in halves)

- 2 celery stalks (chopped or sliced thinly)

- ½ cup arugula

- ½ small red onion (diced)

- 2 Medjool pitted dates (chopped)

- 1 tbsp. of dark chocolate powder

- 1 tbsp. extra virgin olive oil

- 2 tbsp. water

- 5 sprigs of parsley (chopped)

- Dash of salt

Directions:

1. In a food processor, blend the dates, chocolate powder, oil, water, and salt. Add the chili and process further. Rub this paste onto the chicken breast, and set it aside, in the refrigerator.

2. Prepare other salad mixings, vegetables, and herbs in a bowl and toss.

3. Cook the chicken in a dash of oil in a pan, until done, about 10-15 minutes over a medium burner.

4. When done, let cool and lay over the salad bed, and serve.

Nutrition: calories 112, fat 5, fiber 4, carbs 5, protein 4

29. Honey Chili Nuts

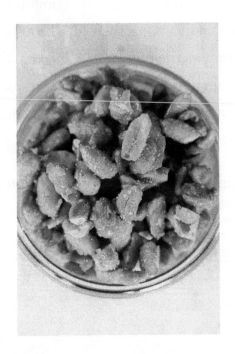

Preparation Time: 10 minutes

Cooking Time: 30 minutes

Servings: 4

Ingredients:

- 5oz walnuts

- 5oz pecan nuts

- 2oz softened butter

- 1 tablespoon honey

- ½ birds-eye chili (very finely chopped and deseeded)

Directions:

1. Preheat the oven to 180°C/360°F. Combine the butter, honey, and chili in a bowl, then add the nuts and stir them well. Spread the nuts onto a lined baking sheet and roast them in the oven for 10 minutes, stirring once halfway through. Remove from the oven and allow them to cool before eating.

Nutrition: calories 62, fat 2, fiber 4, carbs 5, protein 2

30.   Cauliflower Nachos

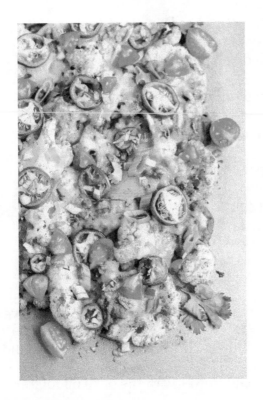

Preparation Time: 5 minutes

Cooking Time: 30 minutes

Servings: 1-2

Ingredients:

- 2 tablespoons extra virgin olive oil

- ½ teaspoon onion powder

- ½ teaspoon turmeric

- ½ teaspoon ground cumin

- 1 medium head cauliflower

- ¾ cup shredded cheddar cheese

- ½ cup tomato (diced)

- ¼ cup red bell pepper (diced)

- ¼ cup red onion (diced)

- ½ Bird's Eye chili pepper (finely diced)

- ¼ cup parsley (finely diced)

- Pinch of salt

Directions:

1. Preheat oven to 400°F.

2. Mix onion powder, cumin, turmeric, and olive oil.

3. Core cauliflower and slice into ½" thick rounds.

4. Coat the cauliflower with the olive oil mixture and bake for 15 – 20 minutes.

5. Top with shredded cheese & bake for an additional 3 – 5 minutes, until cheese is melted.

6. In a bowl, combine tomatoes, bell pepper, onion, chili, and parsley with a pinch of salt.

7. Top cooked cauliflower with salsa and serve.

Nutrition: calories 112, fat 5, fiber 4, carbs 5, protein 4

31. Tofu Smoothie

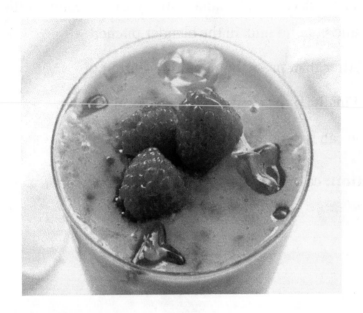

Preparation Time: 5 minutes

Cooking Time: 5 Minutes

Servings: 2 Servings

Ingredients:

- 1 Banana, sliced & frozen

- 3/4 cup Almond Milk

- 2 tbsp. Peanut Butter

- 1/2 cup Yoghurt (plain & low-fat)

- 1/2 cup Tofu (soft & silken)

- 1/3 cup Dates (chopped)

Directions:

1. First, place tofu, banana, dates, yogurt, peanut butter, and almond milk in the blender pitcher.

2. After that, press the 'smoothie' button.

3. Finally, transfer to serving glass and enjoy it.

Tip: You can try adding herbs to your preference.

Nutrition: calories 119, fat 2, fiber 4, carbs 5, protein 4

32.   Grape Smoothie

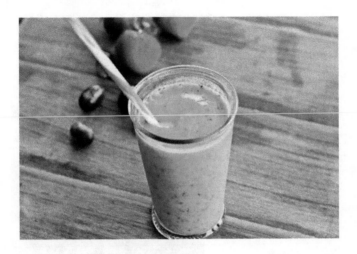

Preparation Time: 5 minutes

Cooking Time: 0 minutes

Servings: 1

Ingredients:

- 2 cups red seedless grapes

- ¼ cup fruit juice

- ½ cup plain yogurt

- 1 cup ice

Directions:

1. Add fruit juice to the blender. At that time, put in the yogurt and grapes. Add the ice last. Blend until smooth, and enjoy!

Nutrition: calories 160, fat 5, fiber 2, carbs 5, protein 3

33.   Kale and Cucumber Smoothie

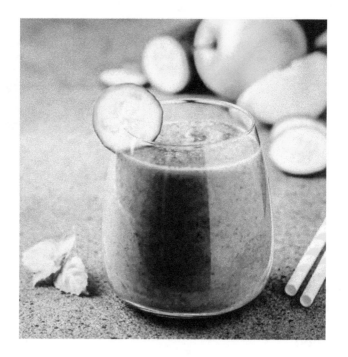

Preparation Time: 5 minutes

Cooking Time: 0 minutes

Servings: 1

Ingredients:

- 1 handful kale

- 2-inch cucumber – sliced (chopped)

- Half-squeezed lime

- 1 medium mango (peeled & chopped)

- 1 tablespoon goji berries

- Extra Water – optionally added to dilute the consistency

Directions:

1. Place all ingredients together in a blender and blend thoroughly.

2. Serve chilled and enjoy!

Nutrition: calories 112, fat 5, fiber 4, carbs 5, protein 4

34.   Mozzarella Cauliflower Bars

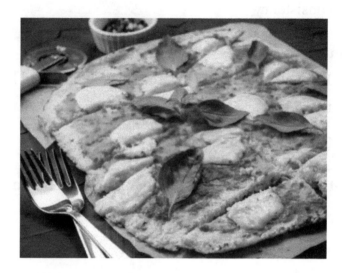

Preparation Time: 10 minutes

Cooking Time: 40 minutes

Servings: 1

Ingredients:

- ½ cauliflower head, riced

- 1/3 cup low-fat mozzarella cheese (shredded)

- ¼ cup egg whites

- 1 teaspoon Italian dressing (low fat)

- Pepper to taste

Directions:

1. Spread cauliflower rice over a lined baking sheet.

2. Preheat your oven to 375°F.

3. Roast for 20 minutes.

4. Transfer to a bowl and spread pepper, cheese, seasoning, egg whites, and stir well.

5. Spread in a rectangular pan and press.

6. Transfer to oven and cook for 20 minutes more.

7. Serve and enjoy!

Nutrition: calories 90, fat 5, fiber 4, carbs 5, protein 4

35.   Walnut and Date Bites

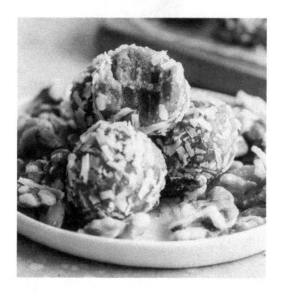

Preparation Time: 5 minutes

Cooking Time: 0 minutes

Servings: 1

Ingredients:

- 3 walnut halves

- 3 pitted Medjool dates

- the ground cinnamon (to taste)

Directions:

1. Cut each walnut carefully into three slices, and do the same with dates. Put a slice of walnut, brush with cinnamon, and serve.

Nutrition: calories 80, fat 7, fiber 41, carbs 3, protein 1

36.   Sirt Energy Balls

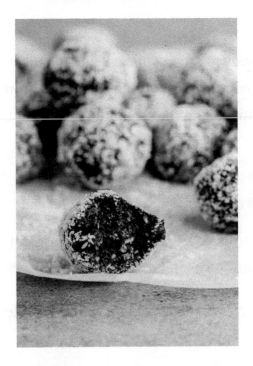

Preparation Time: 5 minutes

Cooking Time: 5 minutes

Servings: 2-4

Ingredients:

- 1 cup old fashion ginger, dried

- 1/4 cup quinoa cooked using 3/4 cup orange juice

- 1/4 cup shredded unsweetened coconut

- 1/3 cup dried cranberry/raisin blend

- 1/3 cup dark chocolate chips

- 1/4 cup slivered almonds

- 1 tbsp. reduced-fat peanut butter

Directions:

1. Cook quinoa in orange juice. Bring to boil and simmer for approximately 1-2 minutes. Let cool. Combine chilled quinoa and the remaining ingredients into a bowl.

2. With wet hands, combine ingredients and roll in golden ball sized chunks.

3. Set at a Tupperware and set in the refrigerator for two weeks until the firm.

Nutrition: calories 82, fat 8, fiber 4, carbs 5, protein 3

37.   Hot Chicory & Nut Salad

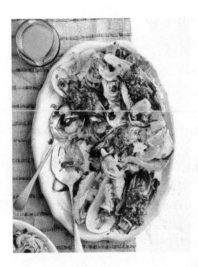

Preparation time: 5 Minutes

Cooking Time: 40 Minutes

Servings: 2

Ingredients:

For the salad:

- 100g 3½oz green beans

- 100g 3½oz red chicory (chopped if unavailable use yellow chicory)

- 100g 3½oz celery (chopped)

- 25g 1oz macadamia nuts (chopped)

- 25g 1oz walnuts (chopped)

- 25g 1oz plain peanuts (chopped)

- 2 tomatoes (chopped)

- 1 tablespoon olive oil

For the dressing:

- 2 tablespoons fresh parsley (finely chopped)

- ½ teaspoon turmeric

- ½ teaspoon mustard

- 1 tablespoon olive oil

- 25mls 1fl oz. red wine vinegar

Directions:

1. Mix the ingredients for the dressing, and then set them aside. Heat a tablespoon of olive oil in a frying pan then add the green beans, chicory, and celery.

2. Cook until the vegetables have softened then add in the chopped tomatoes and cook for 2 minutes.

3. Add the prepared dressing, and thoroughly coat all of the vegetables. Serve onto plates and sprinkle the mixture of nuts over the top. Eat immediately.

Nutrition: calories 438, fat 5, fiber 4, carbs 13, protein 54

38. Tuscan Bean Stew

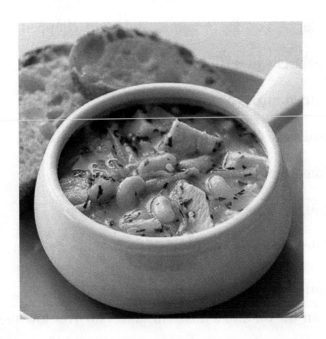

Preparation Time: 20 minutes

Cooking Time: 15 minutes

Servings: 2

Ingredients:

- 1 Chopped Italian Tomatoes

- 1.5 ounces Buckwheat

- 1 tablespoon Extra virgin olive oil

- Vegetable stock - 200ml

- Red onion - ¾ cup (finely chopped)

- Carrot – ¼ cup (peeled and finely chopped)

- Herbes de Provence - 1 teaspoon

- Celery – 1 ounce (trimmed and finely chopped)

- Garlic clove - 1 (finely chopped)

- Tinned mixed beans – 1 cup

- Bird's eye chili - ½ (finely chopped), optional

- Tomato purée - 1 teaspoon

- Roughly chopped parsley - 1 tablespoon

- Kale – ½ cup (roughly chopped)

Directions:

1. Pour the oil into a medium saucepan over low-medium heat. Once hot, add the onion, celery, carrot, herbs, garlic, and chili and stir fry until the onion gets soft but not colored.

2. Add the tomatoes, stock, and the tomato puree to the pan and bring to a boil. Add the beans and allow to simmer for 30 minutes.

3. Add the kale and cook for an additional 5 to 10 minutes, until tender. Now add the parsley.

4. In the casserole cook the buckwheat following the directions on the packet. Drain the water, then serve with the stew

Nutrition: calories 112, fat 5, fiber 4, carbs 5, protein 4

39. Sirtfood Cauliflower Couscous and Turkey Steak

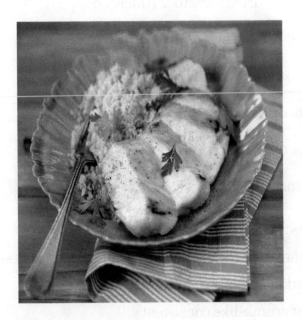

Preparation Time: 45 minutes

Cooking Time: 10 minutes

Servings: 2

Ingredients:

- 5 ¼ oz. cauliflower (roughly chopped)

- 1 garlic clove (finely chopped)

- 1 ½ oz. red onion (finely chopped)

- 1 bird's eye chili (finely chopped)

- 1 tsp. finely chopped fresh ginger

- 2 tbsp. extra virgin olive oil

- 2 tsp. ground turmeric

- 1 oz. sun-dried tomatoes (finely chopped)

- ⅜ oz. parsley

- 5 ¼ oz. turkey steak

- 1 tsp. dried sage

- Juice of ½ lemon

- 1 tbsp. capers

Directions:

1. Disintegrate the cauliflower using a food processor. Blend in 1-2 pulses until the cauliflower has a breadcrumb-like consistency.

2. In a skillet, fry garlic, chili, ginger, and red onion in 1 tsp. olive oil for 2-3 minutes. Throw in the turmeric and cauliflower, and then cook for another 1-2 minutes. Remove from heat and add the tomatoes and roughly half the parsley.

3. Garnish the turkey steak with sage and dress with oil. In a skillet, over medium heat, fry the turkey steak for 5 minutes, turning occasionally. Once the steak is cooked add lemon juice, capers, and a dash of water. Stir and serve with the couscous.

Nutrition: calories 452, fat 39, fiber 4, carbs 10, protein 15

---

40. Chicken Thighs with Tomato Spinach Sauce

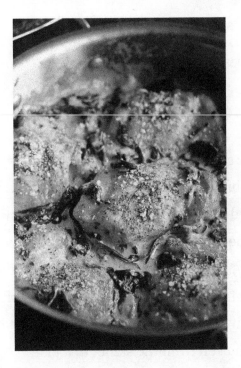

Preparation Time: 45 minutes

Cooking Time: 10 minutes

Servings: 2

Ingredients:

- 1 tablespoon olive oil

- 1.5 lb. chicken thighs (boneless skinless)

- ½ teaspoon salt

- ¼ teaspoon pepper

- 8 oz. tomato sauce

- Two garlic cloves (minced)

- ½ cup overwhelming cream

- 4 oz. new spinach

- Four leaves fresh basil (or utilize ¼ teaspoon dried basil)

Directions:

1. The most effective method to cook boneless skinless chicken thighs in a skillet: In a much skillet, heat olive oil on medium warmth. Season boneless chicken with salt and pepper. Add top side down to the hot skillet. Cook for 5 minutes on medium heat, until the high side, is pleasantly burned. Flip over to the opposite side and heat for five additional minutes on medium heat. Take out the chicken from the skillet to a plate.

2. Step by step instructions to make creamy tomato basil sauce: To the equivalent, presently void skillet, include tomato sauce, minced garlic, and substantial cream. Bring to bubble and mix. Lessen warmth to low stew. Include new spinach and new basil.

3. Mix until spinach withers and diminishes in volume. Taste the sauce and include progressively salt and pepper, if necessary. Include back cooked boneless skinless chicken thighs, increment warmth to medium.

Nutrition: calories 602, fat 55, fiber 4, carbs 30, protein 66

41.Chicken with Mole Salad

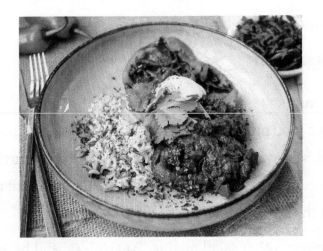

Preparation Time: 5 minutes

Cooking Time: 40 minutes

Servings: 2

Ingredients:

- 1 skinned chicken breast

- 2 cups spinach, washed (dried and torn in halves)

- 2 celery stalks (chopped or sliced thinly)

- ½ cup arugula

- ½ small red onion (diced)

- 2 Medjool pitted dates (chopped)

- 1 tbsp. of dark chocolate powder

- 1 tbsp. extra virgin olive oil

- 2 tbsp. water

- 5 sprigs of parsley (chopped)

- Dash of salt

Directions:

1. In a food processor, blend the dates, chocolate powder, oil, water, and salt. Add the chili and process further. Rub this paste onto the chicken breast, and set it aside, in the refrigerator.

2. Prepare other salad mixings, vegetables, and herbs in a bowl and toss.

3. Cook the chicken in a dash of oil in a pan, until done, about 10-15 minutes over a medium burner.

4. When done, let cool and lay over the salad bed, and serve.

Nutrition: calories 112, fat 5, fiber 4, carbs 5, protein 4

42.   Honey Chili Squash

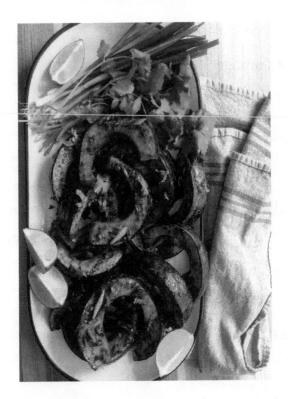

Preparation time: 5 Minutes

Cooking Time: 50 Minutes

Servings: 2

Ingredients:

- 2 red onions, roughly chopped 2.5cm

- 1-inch chunk of ginger root (finely chopped)

- 2 cloves of garlic

- 2 bird's-eye chilies (finely chopped)

- 1 butternut squash (peeled and chopped)

- 100 ml 3½ fl. oz. vegetable stock broth

- 1 tablespoon olive oil

- Juice of 1 orange

- Juice of 1 lime

- 2 teaspoons honey

Directions:

1. Warm the oil into a pan and add in the red onions, squash chunks, chilies, garlic, ginger, and honey.

2. Cook for 3 minutes. Squeeze in the lime and orange juice.

3. Pour in the stock broth, orange, and lime juice and cook for 15 minutes until tender.

Nutrition: calories214, fat 20, fiber 4, carbs 25, protein 11

43. Turkey Escalope with Cauliflower Couscous

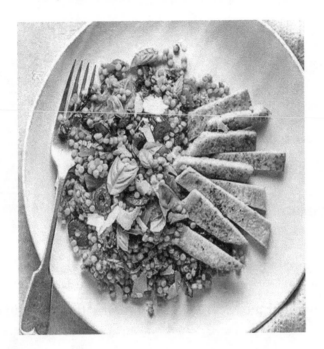

Preparation time: 5 Minutes

Cooking Time: 50 Minutes

Servings: 2

Ingredients:

- 150g cauliflower (roughly chopped)

- 1 clove of garlic (finely chopped)

- 40g red onions (finely chopped)

- 1 Thai chili (finely chopped)

- 1 teaspoon chopped fresh ginger

- 2 tablespoons of extra virgin olive oil

- 2 teaspoons turmeric

- 30g dried tomatoes (finely chopped)

- 10g parsley leaves

- 150g turkey escalope

- 1 teaspoon dried sage

- Juice of a 1/4 lemon

- 1 tablespoon capers

Directions:

1. Mix the cauliflower in a food processor until the individual pieces are slightly smaller than a grain of rice.

2. Heat the garlic, onions, chili, and ginger in a frying pan with a tablespoon of olive oil until they are slightly glazed. Add turmeric and cauliflower mix well and heat for about 1 minute. Then remove from heat and add half of the parsley and all the tomatoes and mix well.

3. Mix the turkey escalope with the oil and sage. Put the rest of the oil in a pan and fry the scallops on both sides until they are ready. Then add the lemon juice, capers, remaining parsley, and a tablespoon of water and warm it up again briefly. Serve with the cauliflower couscous.

Nutrition: calories 282, fat 16, fiber 4, carbs 5, protein 26

44.   Strawberry Arugula Salad

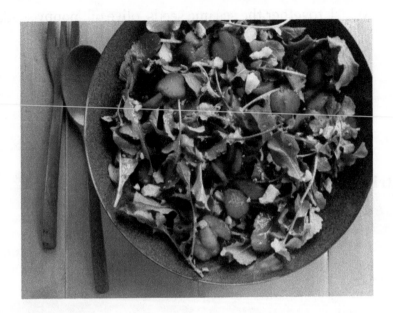

Preparation time: 5 Minutes

Cooking Time: 60 Minutes

Servings: 4-6

Ingredients:

- 2 tbsp. black sesame seeds

- 1 tbsp. poppy seeds

- 1/2 cup olive oil

- 1/4 cup lemon juice

- 1/4 tsp. paprika

- 1 bag fresh arugula (chopped, washed, and dried)

- 1 ½ cup strawberries (sliced)

Directions:

1. Whisk together the sesame seeds, olive oil, poppy seeds, paprika, lemon juice, and onion. Refrigerate.

2. In a large bowl, combine arugula, strawberries, and walnuts. Pour dressing over salad.

3. Toss and refrigerate 15 minutes before serving.

Nutrition: calories 112, fat 5, fiber 4, carbs 5, protein 4

45. Serrano Ham & Rocket Arugula

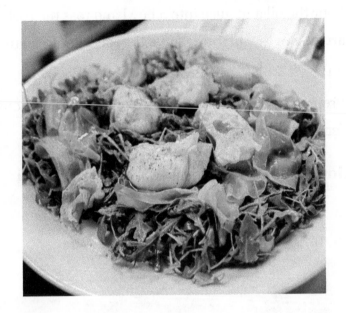

Preparation time: 5 Minutes

Cooking Time: 60 Minutes

Servings: 2

Ingredients:

- 175g 6 oz. Serrano ham

- 125g 4 oz. rocket arugula leaves

- 2 tablespoons olive oil

- 1 tablespoon orange juice

Directions:

1. Pour the oil and juice into a bowl and toss the rocket arugula in the mixture. Serve the rocket onto plates and top it off with the ham.

2. Prepare buckwheat according to package Directions, serve with meat and vegetables.

Nutrition: calories 112, fat 5, fiber 4, carbs 5, protein 4

46.   Tomato & Goat's Cheese Pizza

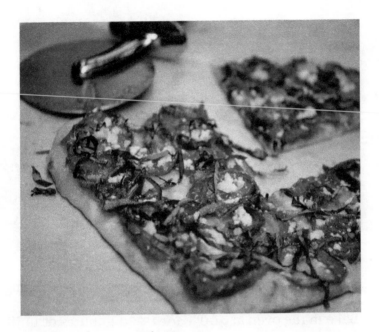

Preparation time: 5 Minutes

Cooking Time: 50 Minutes

Servings: 2

Ingredients:

- 225g 8 oz. buckwheat flour

- 2 teaspoons dried yeast

- Pinch of salt

- 150mls 5fl oz. slightly water

- 1 teaspoon olive oil

- For the Topping:

- 75g 3oz. feta cheese (crumbled)

- 75g 3oz. passata or tomato paste

- 1 tomato (sliced)

- 1 red onion (finely chopped)

- 25g 1oz. rocket arugula leaves (chopped)

Directions:

1. In a bowl, combine all the ingredients for the pizza dough then allow it to stand for at least an hour until it has doubled in size.

2. Roll the dough out to a size to suit you. Spoon the passata onto the base and add the rest of the toppings.

3. Bake in the oven at 400°F for 15-20 minutes or until browned at the edges and crispy and serve.

Nutrition: calories 302, fat 12, fiber 4, carbs 12, protein 9

47.   Banana Dessert

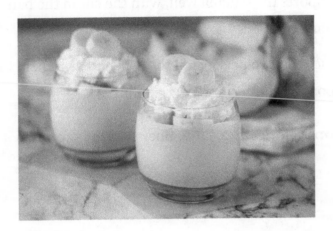

Preparation Time: 15 minutes

Cooking Time: 10 minutes

Servings: 2 - 3

Ingredients:

- 2 pieces Banana (ripe)

- 2 tablespoons pure chocolate (> 70% cocoa)

- 2 tablespoons Almond leaves

Directions:

1. Chop the chocolate finely, cut the banana lengthwise, but not completely, as the banana must serve as a casing for the chocolate.

2. Slightly slide on the banana, spread the finely chopped chocolate and almonds over the bananas.

3. Fold a kind of boat out of the aluminum foil that supports the banana well, with the cut in the banana facing up.

4. Place the two packets on the grill and grill them for about 4 minutes until the skin is dark.

Nutrition: calories 232, fat 2, fiber 2, carbs 5, protein 4

48.   Salad with Roasted Carrots

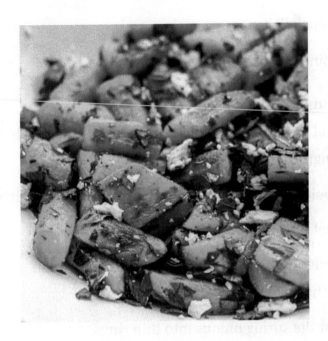

Preparation Time: 10 minutes

Cooking Time: 5 minutes

Servings: 2 - 3

Ingredients:

- 1 hand-mixed salad

- 500g Carrot

- 1 piece Orange

- 100g Pecans

- 1/2 teaspoon dried thyme

- 1 tablespoon Honey

- 1 tablespoon Olive oil

- 1 pinch Salt

- 1 pinch Black pepper

Directions:

1. Peel the carrots and cut the green. Cut them in half lengthways.

2. Cook the carrots al dente for 5 minutes and drain well.

3. Peel the orange and cut it into pieces.

4. Roughly chop the pecans and briefly fry them in a pan without oil.

5. Cut the spring onions into thin rings.

6. Place the carrots in a bowl with 1 tablespoon of olive oil, a pinch of salt and pepper, and the thyme.

7. Roast the carrots briefly on the grill or in a grill pan. Until they have nice grill marks.

8. Mix the salad with carrots and honey and put it on a plate.

9. Spread the orange slices and pecans over the salad.

Nutrition: calories 102, fat 5, fiber 23, carbs 50, protein 15

49. Salmon with Capers and Lemon

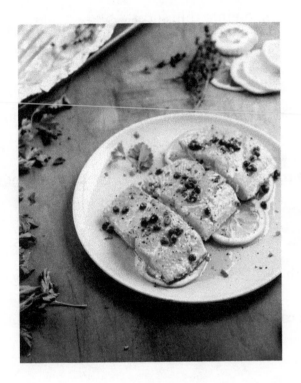

Preparation Time: 10 minutes

Cooking Time: 15 minutes

Servings: 2 - 3

Ingredients:

- 2 pieces salmon fillet

- 1 tablespoon Coconut oil

- 2 tablespoon capers

- 1/2 pieces

Directions:

1. Cut the lemon into thin slices.

2. Take an aluminum tray or piece of aluminum foil that is folded in half.

3. First, layout 4 slices of lemon and spread the capers on them.

4. Place the salmon on the capers. Then put a lemon wedge on the salmon.

5. Fry the salmon on the grill (with aluminum dish/foil).

6. Season with salt and pepper just before serving.

Nutrition: calories 122, fat 14, fiber 1, carbs 2, protein 1

50.   Pasta Salad

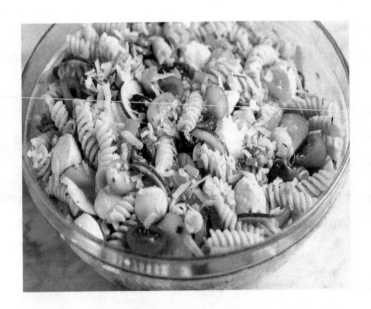

Preparation Time: 15 minutes

Cooking Time: 5 minutes

Servings: 2 - 3

Ingredients:

- 125g green asparagus

- 1 hand Cherry tomatoes

- 1/2 pieces yellow bell pepper

- 1/2 pieces Red bell pepper

- 125g Sesame fusilli

- 3 tablespoon Olive oil

- 1 tablespoon Red wine vinegar

- 1 teaspoon dried oregano

Directions:

1. Cook the sesame fusilli as indicated on the package.

2. After cooking the pasta, drain with cold water.

3. Slice the green asparagus into pieces.

4. Heat a grill pan and grill the asparagus al dente.

5. Cut the cherry tomatoes into pieces; some in halves and some in quarters, this gives the salad a nice playful effect.

6. Cut the two half peppers into long thin strips.

7. Mix the pasta, asparagus, tomatoes, and peppers in a large bowl.

8. Combine the ingredients for the dressing in a small bowl.

9. Stir the dressing through the pasta salad.

Nutrition: calories 112, fat 5, fiber 4, carbs 5, protein 4

51. Pine and Sunflower Seed Rolls

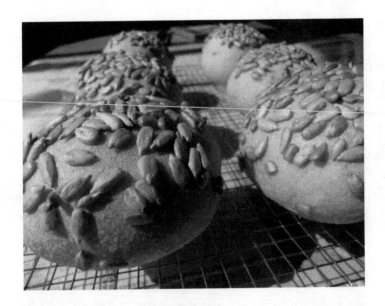

Preparation Time: 20 minutes

Cooking Time: 35 minutes

Servings: 12

Ingredients:

- 120g Tapioca flour

- 1 teaspoon Celtic sea salt

- 4 tablespoon Coconut flour

- 120ml Olive oil

- 120ml Water (warm)

- 1 piece Egg (beaten)

- 150g Pine nuts (roasted)

- 150g Sunflower seeds (roasted)
- Baking paper sheet

Directions:

1. Preheat the oven to 160°C.

2. Put the pine nuts and sunflower seeds in a small bowl and set them aside.

3. Mix the tapioca with the salt and tablespoons of coconut flour in a large bowl. Pour the olive oil and warm water into the mixture.

4. Add the egg and mix until you get an even batter. Add 1 tablespoon of coconut flour at a time until it has the desired consistency if the dough is too thin.

5. Wait a few minutes between each addition of the flour so that it can absorb the moisture. The dough should be soft and sticky.

6. With a wet tablespoon, take tablespoons of batter to make a roll. Put some tapioca flour on your hands so the dough doesn't stick. Fold the dough with your fingertips instead of rolling it in your palms.

7. Place the roll in the bowl of pine nuts and sunflower seeds and roll it around until covered. Line a baking sheet with parchment paper. Place the buns on the

baking sheet. Cook in the preheated oven for 35 minutes and serve warm.

Nutrition: calories 262, fat 70, fiber 24, carbs 54, protein 64

52.   Tofu with Cauliflower

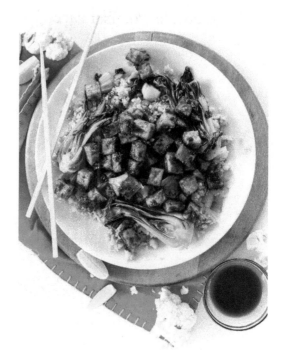

Preparation time: 5 minutes

Cooking time: 45 minutes

Servings: 2

Ingredients:

- ¼ cup red pepper (seeded)

- 1 Thai chili (cut in two halves, seeded)

- 2 cloves of garlic

- 1 tsp. of olive oil

- 1 pinch of cumin

- 1 pinch of coriander

- Juice of a half lemon

- 8 oz. tofu

- 8 oz. cauliflower (roughly chopped)

- 1 ½ oz. red onions (finely chopped)

- 1 tsp. finely chopped ginger

- 2 teaspoons turmeric

- 1 oz. dried tomatoes (finely chopped)

- 1 oz. parsley (chopped)

Directions:

1. Preheat oven to 400°F. Slice the peppers and put them in an ovenproof dish with chili and garlic.

2. Pour some olive oil over it, add the dried herbs, and put it in the oven until the peppers are soft (about 20 minutes).

3. Let it cool down, put the peppers together with the lemon juice in a blender and work it into a soft mass.

4. Cut the tofu in half and divide the halves into triangles.

5. Place the tofu in a small casserole dish, cover with the paprika mixture, and place in the oven for about 20 minutes.

6. Chop the cauliflower until the pieces are smaller than a grain of rice.

7. Then, in a small saucepan, heat the garlic, onions, chili, and ginger with olive oil until they become transparent. Add turmeric and cauliflower mix well and heat again.

8. Remove from heat and add parsley and tomatoes mix well. Serve with the tofu in the sauce.

Nutrition: Calories 29, Fat 5, Carbs 55 g, Protein 27

53.   Sweet and Sour Pan

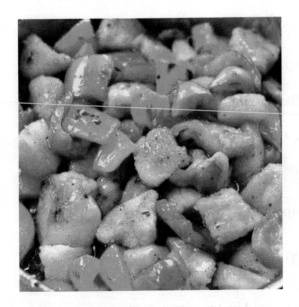

Preparation time: 30 minutes

Cooking time: 0 minutes

Servings: 2

Ingredients:

- 2 tbsp. Coconut oil

- 2 pieces Red onion

- 2 pieces yellow bell pepper

- 12 oz. White cabbage

- 6 oz. Pak choi

- 1 ½ oz. Mung bean sprouts

- 4 Pineapple slices

- 1 ½ oz. Cashew nuts

- ¼ cup Apple cider vinegar

- 4 tbsp. Coconut blossom sugar

- 1½ tbsp. Tomato paste

- 1 tsp. Coconut-Aminos

- 2 tsp. Arrowroot powder

- ¼ cup Water

Directions:

1. Roughly cut the vegetables. Mix the arrowroot with five tbsp. of cold water into a paste.

2. Then put all the other ingredients for the sauce in a saucepan and add the arrowroot paste for binding.

3. Melt the coconut oil in a pan and fry the onion. Add the bell pepper, cabbage, pak choi, and bean sprouts and stir-fry until the vegetables become a little softer.

4. Add the pineapple, cashew nuts, and stir a few more times. Pour a little sauce over the wok dish and serve.

Nutrition: calories 572, fat 27, fiber 4, carbs 89, protein 12

54.   Vegetarian Curry

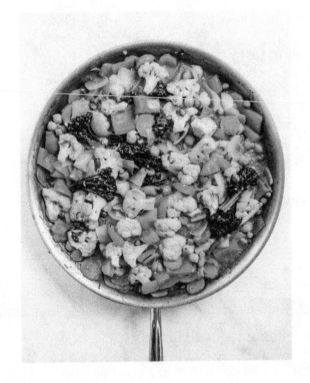

Preparation time: 15 minutes

Cooking time: 60 minutes

Servings: 2

Ingredients:

- 4 medium Carrots

- 2 medium Sweet potatoes

- 1 large Onion

- 3 cloves Garlic

- 4 tbsp. Curry powder

- ½ tsp. caraway (ground)

- ½ tsp. Chili powder

- Sea salt to taste

- 1 pinch Cinnamon

- ½ cup Vegetable broth

- 1 can Tomato cubes

- 8 oz. Sweet peas

- 2 tbsp. Tapioca flour

Directions:

1. Roughly chop carrots, sweet potatoes, onions, and garlic and put them all in a pot.

2. Mix tapioca flour with curry powder, cumin, chili powder, salt, and cinnamon, and sprinkle this mixture on the vegetables.

3. Add tomato cubes. Pour the vegetable broth over it.

4. Close the pot with a lid, bring it to a boil and let it simmer for 60 minutes on low heat. Stir in snap peas after 30min. Cauliflower rice is a great addition to this dish.

Nutrition: calories 112, fat 5, fiber 4, carbs 5, protein 4

55.   Spiced Burger

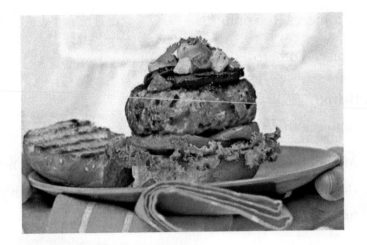

Preparation Time: 20 minutes

Cooking Time: 25 minutes

Servings: 2 - 4

Ingredients:

- Ground beef 250g

- 1 clove Garlic

- 1 teaspoon dried oregano

- 1 teaspoon Paprika powder

- 1 / 2 TL Caraway ground

Toppings:

- 4 pieces Mushrooms

- 1 piece Little Gem

- 1/4 pieces Zucchini

- 1/2 pieces Red onion

- 1 piece Tomato

Directions:

1. Squeeze the clove of garlic.

2. Mix all the ingredients for the burgers in a bowl. Divide the mixture into two halves and crush the halves into hamburgers.

3. Place the burgers on a plate and put them in the fridge for a while.

4. Cut the zucchini diagonally into 1 cm slices.

5. Cut the red onion into half rings. Cut the tomato into thin slices and cut the leaves of the Little Gem salad.

6. Grill the hamburgers on the grill until they're done.

7. Place the mushrooms beside the burgers and grill on both sides until cooked but firm.

8. Place the zucchini slices beside it and grill briefly.

9. Now it's time to build the burger!

10. Place 2 mushrooms on a plate, then stack the lettuce, a few slices of zucchini, and tomatoes. Then put the burger on top and finally add the red onion.

Nutrition: calories 122, fat 2, fiber 7, carbs 25, protein 7